Candida Symptoms

Chapter List:

Book Introduction:

Welcome to "The Silent Battle: Conquering Candida." In this comprehensive guide, we embark on a journey to uncover the truth behind Candida overgrowth and its impact on our physical, mental, and emotional well-being. Candida, a stubborn fungal organism, silently lurks within our bodies, wreaking havoc on our health while often remaining undetected.

Have you ever experienced unexplained fatigue, recurrent yeast infections, or digestive issues? Perhaps you've struggled with brain fog, mood swings, or even stubborn weight gain. These seemingly unrelated symptoms may all be manifestations of Candida overgrowth.

This book serves as your compass in navigating the complex terrain of Candida, offering you insights, strategies, and practical tips to reclaim your health and vitality. From understanding the underlying causes and symptoms to implementing effective treatment protocols, each chapter delves into a crucial aspect of the Candida battle.

But this is not just another medical manual. "The Silent Battle: Conquering Candida" aims to empower you emotionally as well. Throughout the pages, we will delve into the emotional toll that Candida inflicts, providing you with the tools to develop resilience, self-compassion, and a renewed sense of inner strength.

Are you ready to embark on this transformative journey? Let's dive into the first chapter, where we unmask Candida, the hidden intruder, and lay the foundation for our battle against this insidious foe.

Chapter 1: Unmasking Candida: The Hidden Intruder

: 1050

In the shadows of our bodies, a silent intruder lies in wait. Candida, a yeast-like fungus, is a natural inhabitant of our gut. In small amounts, it coexists harmoniously with other microorganisms, supporting our digestion and overall health. However, when the delicate balance is disrupted, Candida seizes the opportunity to proliferate, giving rise to a condition known as Candida overgrowth or candidiasis.

This chapter aims to unravel the mystery surrounding Candida, shedding light on its origins, triggers, and the mechanisms that allow it to wreak havoc within our bodies. By understanding the enemy, we can better equip ourselves for the battle ahead.

Candida has a cunning nature, remaining inconspicuous until it reaches a tipping point. The delicate balance of our gut ecosystem can be disturbed by various factors such as prolonged antibiotic use, a diet high in sugar and refined carbohydrates, chronic stress, hormonal imbalances, and weakened immune function.

As Candida multiplies, it morphs from its benign yeast form into an invasive fungal form, penetrating the gut lining and releasing toxic byproducts into the bloodstream. These toxins trigger an array of symptoms that can manifest throughout the body, affecting multiple systems and organs.

The first signs of Candida overgrowth are often nonspecific, making diagnosis challenging. Fatigue, brain fog, digestive disturbances, and recurrent yeast infections are just a few of the myriad symptoms that may emerge. It is crucial to recognize the interconnectedness of these seemingly unrelated manifestations and consider Candida as a potential underlying cause.

By unmasking Candida and shining a light on its intricate mechanisms, we can empower ourselves to take back control. In the chapters that follow, we will explore the symptoms, complications, and treatment options available to conquer Candida and restore balance to our bodies.

Join us on this journey as we dive deeper into the hidden world of Candida, unlocking the secrets to overcoming its silent reign of havoc.

<u>Stay tuned for Chapter 2: Candida Overgrowth: A System in Chaos. Together, we will uncover the far-reaching effects of Candida overgrowth and discover the path towards</u>

reclaiming our health and vitality.

Chapter 2: Candida Overgrowth: A System in Chaos

: 1025

Emotions run high as we delve into the intricate web woven by Candida overgrowth. It's not just a physical battle but a silent assailant that disrupts the harmony of our entire being. Candida's insidious presence sends shockwaves through our bodies, leaving no system untouched.

Imagine waking up each morning feeling as if you've been drained of life force, your energy reserves depleted. The simplest tasks become arduous challenges, and your vitality fades away like a distant memory. This is the relentless grip of Candida overgrowth, pulling you into a system in chaos.

Digestive disturbances become the norm as Candida wreaks havoc on your gut health. Bloating, gas, constipation, or diarrhea become unwelcome companions on your daily journey. Your gut, once a thriving ecosystem of beneficial bacteria, becomes an arena where Candida dominates, feeding off the sugars and refined carbohydrates you consume.

But the chaos doesn't stop there. Candida's malevolent influence extends to your mental and emotional well-being, clouding your thoughts and emotions like a dense fog. Brain fog descends upon you, causing confusion, difficulty concentrating, and memory lapses. Your once sharp mind feels trapped in a haze, hindering your ability to perform at your best.

The emotional toll of Candida overgrowth can be profound. Anxiety and depression creep into your life, casting a shadow over even the brightest moments. Your emotional landscape becomes a battleground, and the weight of it all feels overwhelming. Yet, remember that you are not alone in this fight. By understanding the emotional aspects of Candida, we can develop resilience and find solace in the knowledge that healing is possible.

Candida's assault on your immune system further intensifies the chaos. Your body's defense mechanisms become compromised, leaving you vulnerable to frequent infections and prolonged illness. The very foundation of your health is shaken, and the journey to restore your immune function becomes an urgent mission.

Hormonal imbalances also fall victim to Candida's influence. Women may experience disrupted menstrual cycles, intense PMS symptoms, or hormonal acne. Men may encounter issues with libido, erectile dysfunction, or unexplained fatigue. The delicate dance of hormones is disrupted, and finding equilibrium becomes an essential part of the healing process.

As we navigate this sea of chaos, it's important to remember that you possess the strength to regain control. While Candida may have thrown your life into disarray, you are resilient. This battle is not without hope. With knowledge, determination, and a willingness to embrace change, you can reclaim your vitality and restore harmony within your body and soul.

In the upcoming chapters, we will explore strategies to conquer Candida and restore balance to your life. From dietary modifications and targeted supplements to lifestyle adjustments and emotional healing, we will arm you with the tools necessary for victory.

Stay with us as we uncover the intricate connections between Candida overgrowth and your overall well-being. In Chapter 3, we will unveil the candid truth behind the symptoms associated with this silent battle. Together, we will forge a path towards a brighter, healthier futureâ€"one free from the shackles of Candida's chaos.

Chapter 3: Candida Symptoms: Unveiling the Silent Battle

: 1003

In the depths of the silent battle with Candida, symptoms become the voice that cries out for recognition. Unveiling these symptoms is like peeling back layers of a complex puzzle, each piece revealing a deeper understanding of the struggle within.

One of the most insidious aspects of Candida is its ability to manifest in various ways, mimicking other conditions and confounding both patients and healthcare professionals. It hides in plain sight, leaving those affected to grapple with a myriad of perplexing symptoms.

Fatigue, the relentless companion of Candida overgrowth, infiltrates every aspect of your life. It drains you physically, mentally, and emotionally, leaving you feeling as if you're wading through quicksand. No matter how much rest you get, the exhaustion persists, a heavy weight upon your shoulders.

But fatigue is not the sole sentinel of this battle. Candida ravages your digestive system, causing symptoms that range from bothersome to debilitating. Bloating distends your abdomen, causing discomfort and an unwelcome self-consciousness. Gas, cramping, and irregular bowel movements disrupt your daily routine, leaving you feeling at odds with your own body.

Recurrent yeast infections, a telltale sign of Candida overgrowth, cast a shadow on your intimate relationships. The itch, the discomfort, the constant battle against an unrelenting foeâ€"it takes a toll on your self-esteem and can strain the bonds with your partner. Candida seeks to isolate you, to erode your confidence, but you are not alone.

Skin issues become a visible battleground, as Candida-related rashes and fungal infections emerge. From stubborn acne and eczema to relentless itching and redness, your skin bears the brunt of this silent struggle. It becomes a canvas marked by the unseen battle within, a reflection of the chaos that lies beneath the surface.

As the battle wages on, your mood becomes a casualty. Candida overgrowth has the power to alter brain chemistry, leading to emotional imbalances that may manifest as anxiety, depression, irritability, or mood swings. You may feel like you're on an emotional rollercoaster, struggling to find stable ground amidst the turbulence.

Weight issues become a source of frustration and confusion. Despite your best efforts, shedding pounds becomes an uphill battle. Candida's influence on your metabolism and hormone regulation disrupts your body's ability to maintain a healthy weight, compounding the emotional toll of this silent battle.

But take heart, for within these symptoms lies the roadmap to your recovery. By understanding the manifestations of Candida overgrowth, you gain the power to take targeted action. Through dietary modifications, antifungal treatments, and holistic approaches, you can restore balance and reclaim your well-being.

This book serves as a guiding light, illuminating the path towards healing and offering you a lifeline amidst the chaos. With each chapter, we delve deeper into the intricacies of this silent battle, arming you with knowledge and empathy to face Candida head-on.

In Chapter 4, we will explore the intimate connection between Candida and digestive health. By understanding how Candida disrupts the

delicate balance of your gut, you will be equipped to take the necessary steps to restore harmony within. Remember, you are not defined by the symptoms you experience. Your strength and resilience will carry you forward on the journey towards conquering Candida and reclaiming your vitality.

Chapter 4: The Gut Connection: Candida and Digestive Health

: 1021

In the intricate dance of health and harmony, the gut takes center stage. It is the epicenter of our well-being, the gateway to vitality. But when Candida infiltrates this sacred space, chaos ensues, and the delicate balance is disrupted.

The gutâ€"a complex ecosystem of trillions of microorganismsâ€"thrives on symbiosis. Beneficial bacteria work tirelessly to support our digestion, nutrient absorption, and immune function. But when Candida seizes the opportunity to overgrow, it becomes a disruptive force, throwing the entire system into disarray.

Candida's insidious nature allows it to exploit weaknesses within the gut environment. Prolonged antibiotic use, a diet high in sugar and refined carbohydrates, chronic stress, hormonal imbalances, and weakened immune function all create an environment ripe for Candida overgrowth.

As Candida flourishes, it morphs from its benign yeast form into an invasive fungal form. It pierces the gut lining, compromising its integrity and causing a condition known as "leaky gut." This breach allows toxins, undigested food particles, and Candida itself to infiltrate the bloodstream, triggering a cascade of inflammatory responses throughout the body.

The digestive symptoms of Candida overgrowth are relentless. Bloating, gas, and abdominal pain become constant companions, a constant reminder of the disruption within. You may find yourself caught in a cycle of fluctuating bowel movementsâ€"constipation followed by bouts of diarrheaâ€"leaving you feeling off-kilter and disconnected from your own body.

But the gut connection goes beyond physical discomfort. Candida's influence extends to your mental and emotional well-being. The gut-brain axis, a bidirectional communication system, links your gut and your brain. When Candida wreaks havoc in your gut, it can disrupt this communication, leading to brain fog, difficulty concentrating, and mood disturbances.

Imagine feeling trapped in a foggy haze, unable to think clearly or find the mental clarity you once possessed. Your ability to focus wanes, leaving you frustrated and doubting your own capabilities. This mental turmoil adds an extra layer of emotional strain to an already challenging battle.

As we embark on the journey to restore digestive health, we must address the root causes of Candida overgrowth. By adopting an anti-Candida diet, we starve the fungus of its primary fuelâ€"sugar and refined carbohydrates. Instead, we nourish our bodies with whole, nutrient-dense foods that support a thriving gut environment.

In addition to dietary modifications, antifungal treatments play a vital role in reclaiming balance. Natural remedies such as herbal supplements, essential oils, and probiotics can help combat Candida overgrowth and restore harmony to your gut.

Healing the gut requires a holistic approachâ€"one that encompasses not only dietary and medicinal interventions but also stress management, adequate sleep, and mindful practices. By embracing a comprehensive plan, you can rebuild the foundation of your health, brick by brick, until your gut becomes a sanctuary of vitality once more.

Remember, dear reader, that your gut is the epicenter of your well-being. The battle against Candida begins here. With each step you take to restore digestive health, you forge a path toward reclaiming your vitality, one that will lead you to a brighter, healthier future.

In Chapter 5, we will explore the intricate relationship between Candida and sugar addiction—a connection that fuels the silent battle within. Brace yourself, for the journey ahead will challenge you to confront your relationship with sweetness and pave the way to a life free from Candida's grip.

Chapter 5: Breaking the Sweet Shackles: Candida and Sugar Addiction

: 1008

In a world dominated by sugary temptations, our taste buds yearn for sweetness, while Candida silently feeds off our desires. The connection between Candida overgrowth and sugar addiction is a vicious cycle—a dance that keeps us captive, shackled to a detrimental habit that fuels the silent battle within.

Sugar addiction is not a mere craving; it is a biochemical response that hijacks our brain's reward system. The allure of sugary treats becomes irresistible, and we find ourselves trapped in a cycle of indulgence, guilt, and the insatiable longing for more. But little do we realize that this very craving is what nourishes the Candida overgrowth, perpetuating the chaos within.

Candida thrives on sugar, transforming it into the energy it needs to multiply and invade our bodies further. The more we indulge in sugar-laden delights, the more Candida prospers, wreaking havoc on our health and amplifying the battle we face.

But breaking free from the sweet shackles is not an easy task. It requires unwavering determination, a shift in mindset, and a deep understanding of the intricate web that connects our sugar cravings to Candida's relentless growth.

As we embark on this journey, we must confront our relationship with sweetness. Sugar has become an omnipresent force in our lives, woven into the fabric of our celebrations, comfort, and even our daily rituals. It is deeply intertwined with our emotions, offering temporary solace and pleasure. Yet, it is this very sweetness that allows Candida to thrive.

The first step towards liberation is awareness. By recognizing the detrimental effects of sugar on our health and understanding the symbiotic relationship between Candida and sugar addiction, we empower ourselves to make informed choices.

Emotional resilience becomes the cornerstone of our journey. Candida and sugar addiction have woven a complex tapestry of emotions within us. The comfort and momentary relief that sugar provides can mask deeper emotional needs, leaving us trapped in a cycle of seeking external gratification. By acknowledging and addressing these emotional aspects, we can break free from the grip of sugar and reclaim our inner strength.

Dietary modifications play a pivotal role in severing the connection between Candida and sugar. An anti-Candida diet involves reducing or eliminating sugars, refined carbohydrates, and processed foods from our daily intake. Instead, we nourish our bodies with whole, nutrient-dense foods that support healing, restore balance, and starve Candida of its primary fuel.

But this journey is not just about restriction; it is about embracing a new relationship with food. We explore the vibrant world of natural sweetness, savoring the flavors of fresh fruits, stevia, or small amounts of healthier alternatives like raw honey or maple syrup. We learn to appreciate the subtle sweetness that nature provides without fueling the Candida fire.

Breaking free from sugar addiction is not a solitary battle. We draw strength from support systemsâ€"family, friends, and even online communitiesâ€"where we can share our triumphs and challenges. Together, we encourage and uplift one another as we navigate the path towards liberation.

Dear reader, as you embark on this transformative journey, remember that the power to break the sweet shackles lies within you. It is not just a battle against Candida; it is a battle for your well-being, your vitality, and your freedom.

In Chapter 6, we dive deeper into the emotional aspects of sugar addiction, uncovering the hidden layers of our cravings and discovering strategies to nurture ourselves without succumbing to the allure

of sugar. Prepare to unearth the strength within and embark on a path towards a life unburdened by Candida's grip and the shackles of sugar addiction.

Chapter 6: Nurturing the Soul: Embracing Self-Care in the Battle Against Sugar Addiction

: 1042

In the midst of the battle against Candida and the stronghold of sugar addiction, self-care emerges as a beacon of light—a lifeline to nourish our souls and guide us towards healing. As we navigate the treacherous terrain of cravings and emotional struggles, it is essential to embrace self-care as an integral part of our journey.

Self-care is not a luxury; it is a vital necessity in our battle against Candida and sugar addiction. It encompasses the practices and rituals that replenish our physical, mental, and emotional well-being, providing the support and resilience we need to overcome the challenges that lie ahead.

At the core of self-care lies self-compassion—a gentle reminder that we are human, imperfect beings deserving of love and care. It is in this space of self-compassion that we find the strength to forgive ourselves for past indulgences and mistakes. We let go of guilt and shame, replacing them with kindness and understanding. Through self-compassion, we create a fertile ground for growth and transformation.

One of the pillars of self-care is nourishing our bodies with wholesome, nutrient-dense foods. As we break free from the grip of sugar addiction, we explore the abundance of natural, unprocessed ingredients that support our health and vitality. We savor the flavors of vibrant vegetables, nourishing fats, and high-quality proteins that fuel our bodies and heal our inner ecosystem.

Movement becomes a form of self-care—a celebration of our bodies' strength and resilience. Engaging in physical activities that bring us joyâ€"whether it's dancing, yoga, or a leisurely walk in natureâ€"releases endorphins, elevates our mood, and helps to alleviate stress. Movement not only supports our physical well-being but also becomes a powerful tool to overcome emotional hurdles.

Mental and emotional self-care become essential in unraveling the deep-seated connection between our emotions and sugar addiction. We cultivate mindfulness and awareness, allowing ourselves to fully experience our thoughts, emotions, and cravings without judgment. Through mindfulness practices such as meditation, deep breathing, and journaling, we develop a greater understanding of the underlying emotions that drive our sugar cravings.

In the realm of self-care, self-expression takes center stage. Engaging in creative activities that bring us joy—such as painting, writing, or playing a musical instrument—provides an outlet for our emotions and fosters a sense of fulfillment. It allows us to express ourselves authentically and connect with the depths of our being.

Social connections form the tapestry of our support system. Surrounding ourselves with positive, uplifting individuals who understand and empathize with our journey is crucial. They become our cheerleaders, offering encouragement, accountability, and a listening ear when we need it the most. Together, we build a community that thrives on mutual support and shared experiences.

Rest and rejuvenation become non-negotiable in our quest for self-care. Creating space for adequate sleep, relaxation, and leisure activities allows our bodies and minds to recharge. We release the notion of constant productivity and embrace the art of slowing down, honoring our need for rest as an act of self-love.

Dear reader, as you embark on this path of self-care, remember that it is not selfish; it is an act of survival. By nurturing your own well-being, you equip yourself with the strength and resilience needed to conquer Candida and overcome sugar addiction. You deserve this investment in yourself.

In Chapter 7, we explore the transformative power

of gratitude and positive affirmations in rewiring our mindset and supporting our journey towards freedom. Brace yourself, for the realm of self-care expands further, opening doors to profound shifts in our perspective and paving the way for lasting change.

Chapter 7: The Power of Gratitude: Harnessing Positivity on the Path to Freedom

: 1006

In the darkest moments of our battle against Candida and sugar addiction, gratitude emerges as a radiant light—a force that has the power to transform our perspective and ignite the flames of positivity. As we navigate the challenges and setbacks, embracing gratitude becomes an essential tool on our path to freedom.

Gratitude is not just a fleeting emotion; it is a practice—a conscious choice to shift our focus towards the blessings that surround us. It is a gentle reminder that even amidst the chaos, there is still goodness and beauty to be found. By cultivating gratitude, we unlock the power to reframe our experiences and find strength in the face of adversity.

In the depths of sugar addiction, it is easy to succumb to feelings of self-pity, frustration, and despair. We may become trapped in a cycle of negativity, fixating on what we perceive as limitations or failures. But through the practice of gratitude, we learn to shift our attention to what is going right, however small it may seem.

Each day, take a moment to reflect on the blessings in your life. It could be the support of loved ones, the beauty of nature, or even the simple joys of everyday lifeâ€"a warm cup of tea, a gentle breeze, or a heartfelt conversation. By intentionally acknowledging and appreciating these moments, we infuse our journey with positivity and resilience.

Gratitude becomes a shield against the onslaught of negative emotions. It reframes our perspective and helps us find meaning in the challenges we face. Rather than viewing setbacks as insurmountable obstacles, we recognize them as opportunities for growth and self-discovery. We learn to be grateful for the lessons they bring and the strength they cultivate within us.

Practicing gratitude also extends to the relationship we have with ourselves. In moments of self-doubt or frustration, we turn inward and acknowledge the progress we have made. We celebrate the small victories—the moments of self-control, the healthy choices, and the self-compassion we offer ourselves. By recognizing our efforts and achievements, we cultivate a deep sense of self-worth and empowerment.

Positive affirmations become a powerful tool in harnessing the energy of gratitude. By consciously affirming positive statements about ourselves and our journey, we reprogram our subconscious mind and shift our beliefs towards a more supportive and uplifting narrative. Affirmations such as "I am strong," "I am worthy of healing," and "I am making progress every day" become anchors of hope and encouragement.

The practice of gratitude extends beyond our own journey. Expressing gratitude to those who support usâ€"family, friends, healthcare providers, or members of our support communityâ€"deepens our connections and fosters a sense of appreciation. It strengthens the bonds of empathy and reminds us that we are not alone in this battle. Gratitude becomes a thread that weaves a tapestry of connection and support.

In moments of temptation or craving, gratitude acts as a powerful anchor. By focusing on the reasons why we embarked on this journeyâ€"the desire for vibrant health, the longing for freedom from Candida's gripâ€"we reconnect with our deepest motivations. We remind ourselves of the incredible resilience and determination that reside within us.

Dear reader, as you embrace the practice of gratitude, remember that it is not a mere platitude; it is a transformative force. It has the power to shift your perspective, ignite your spirit, and infuse your journey with positivity and resilience. By harnessing the power of gratitude, you pave the way for a future where freedom from Candida and sugar addiction becomes your reality.

In Chapter 8, we delve into the realm of mindfulness—a powerful tool that allows us to be present, observe our thoughts and cravings with compassion, and make conscious choices that align with our well-being. Prepare to explore the art of mindfulness and

discover how it can guide you towards a life of liberation and inner peace.

Chapter 8: The Art of Mindfulness: Cultivating Presence Amidst the Chaos

: 1003

In the midst of the chaotic battle against Candida and sugar addiction, mindfulness emerges as a gentle refuge—a sanctuary where we can find solace and reclaim our inner peace. In a world filled with distractions and noise, the practice of mindfulness invites us to anchor ourselves in the present moment and cultivate a deep sense of awareness.

Mindfulness is not just a passing trend; it is an ancient art—a way of being that has the power to transform our relationship with ourselves and the world around us. It is the practice of paying attention, non-judgmentally, to the present moment, inviting us to observe our thoughts, emotions, and cravings with curiosity and compassion.

Amidst the whirlwind of cravings and emotional triggers, mindfulness becomes our guiding light. It allows us to pause, take a breath, and consciously choose our response instead of reacting impulsively. Through mindfulness, we recognize the subtle cues and sensations in our bodies, empowering us to make choices that honor our well-being.

In the realm of food, mindfulness invites us to savor each bite, to engage all our senses in the act of nourishment. By eating mindfully, we become attuned to the signals of hunger and fullness, allowing us to make conscious decisions about what and how much to eat. We liberate ourselves from mindless eating and find a deeper appreciation for the nourishment that sustains us.

Mindfulness also extends to the realm of emotions. It invites us to observe our cravings without judgment, acknowledging them as transient experiences that arise and fade away. By cultivating a compassionate stance towards our emotions, we create space for self-understanding and self-compassion. We learn to respond to our cravings with kindness and explore healthier alternatives to meet our emotional needs.

Through mindfulness, we develop a greater understanding of the intricate web of triggers that contribute to our sugar cravings. We become aware of the external influencesâ€"the advertising, social pressures, and environmental cuesâ€"that fuel our desires. With this awareness, we gain the power to make conscious choices that align with our long-term well-being, untangling ourselves from the grip of mindless consumption.

The practice of mindfulness extends beyond the realm of food and cravings. It permeates every aspect of our lives, allowing us to be fully present in each moment. Mindfulness guides us to find joy in the simple pleasures—a warm ray of sunlight, the melody of birdsong, or the gentle touch of a loved one. It invites us to slow down, to savor the richness of life, and to find gratitude for the precious moments that often go unnoticed.

In the battle against Candida and sugar addiction, mindfulness becomes an anchor amidst the storm—a steady presence that reminds us of our inner strength and resilience. It teaches us to embrace the present moment, with all its challenges and uncertainties, and to trust in our ability to navigate the journey ahead.

Dear reader, as you embark on the path of mindfulness, remember that it is not a destination but a lifelong practice. It is a gift you give yourselfâ€"a tool that empowers you to reclaim your inner peace, cultivate self-awareness, and make conscious choices that support your well-being.

In Chapter 9, we delve into the realm of self-compassionâ€"a vital aspect of our healing journey. Prepare to discover the transformative power of self-compassion and how it can nurture your soul as you continue to navigate the labyrinth of Candida and sugar addiction.

Chapter 9: The Healing Power of Self-Compassion: Nurturing Your Soul in the Midst of the Battle

: 1011

In the midst of the relentless battle against Candida and sugar addiction, self-compassion emerges as a healing balm—a gentle embrace that soothes our weary souls and reminds us of our inherent worthiness. As we navigate the labyrinth of challenges and setbacks, cultivating self-compassion becomes an essential practice on our path to healing.

Self-compassion is not an indulgence; it is a profound act of love and kindness towards ourselves. It is the practice of treating ourselves with the same care and understanding we would offer to a dear friend in need. It is a powerful antidote to the harsh self-judgment and criticism that often accompany our struggles with Candida and sugar addiction.

In moments of temptation or perceived failures, self-compassion invites us to extend grace to ourselves. Instead of berating ourselves for slipping up or succumbing to cravings, we embrace our humanness and offer ourselves forgiveness. We recognize that setbacks are part of the journey and that our worthiness is not defined by our ability to be perfect.

Self-compassion creates a safe space for healing and growth. It allows us to acknowledge the pain and challenges we have faced without judgment or resistance. We offer ourselves the support and empathy we need to navigate the complexities of our emotions, allowing them to be felt and processed with tenderness. Through self-compassion, we honor our vulnerabilities and nurture our inner resilience.

At the core of self-compassion lies self-careâ€"an unwavering commitment to our well-being. We prioritize our physical, emotional, and mental needs, understanding that self-care is not a luxury but a vital component of our healing journey. We create boundaries that protect our energy, engage in activities that bring us joy and relaxation, and surround ourselves with people who uplift and support us.

Self-compassion also invites us to challenge the harsh beliefs and narratives we may hold about ourselves. It asks us to question the self-critical thoughts that undermine our self-worth and replace them with affirming and empowering statements. We cultivate a loving and compassionate inner dialogue—one that recognizes our strengths, acknowledges our efforts, and celebrates our progress.

In the realm of relationships, self-compassion transforms the way we interact with others. It allows us to set healthy boundaries and prioritize our needs without guilt or self-doubt. We learn to communicate our desires and limitations with kindness and assertiveness, fostering relationships that honor and nourish our well-being. By valuing ourselves, we attract individuals who appreciate and respect us.

Self-compassion extends to our bodies—the very vessels that carry us through life's challenges. Instead of fixating on perceived flaws or comparing ourselves to unrealistic ideals, we embrace our bodies with love and gratitude. We nourish ourselves with wholesome foods, engage in movement that brings us joy, and cultivate a sense of appreciation for the incredible resilience and beauty that resides within us.

Dear reader, as you embark on the path of self-compassion,

remember that you are worthy of love, understanding, and healing. Embrace your imperfections, honor your journey, and offer yourself the kindness and compassion you deserve. In moments of doubt or struggle, remember that self-compassion is not a sign of weakness but a profound act of courage and resilience.

In Chapter 10, we delve into the power of community and connectionâ€"a vital aspect of our healing journey. Get ready to discover the strength and support that can be found in the bonds we create with others as we

Chapter 10: Embracing Community: Finding Strength in Connection

: 1009

In the arduous battle against Candida and sugar addiction, community emerges as a lifelineâ€"a source of strength and understanding that can light our path and carry us through the darkest moments. As we navigate the intricate landscape of healing, embracing community becomes a transformative aspect of our journey.

Community is not merely a gathering of individuals; it is a tapestry of shared experiences, empathy, and support. It is a reminder that we are not alone in our struggles—that there are others who understand the challenges we face and offer a helping hand or a listening ear. In community, we find solace and belonging.

Connecting with others who share similar journeys creates a space of understanding and validation. It offers a sanctuary where we can share our triumphs, setbacks, and everything in between without fear of judgment. In this safe space, we find encouragement, inspiration, and the courage to keep moving forward.

The power of community lies not only in the support it provides but also in the wisdom and knowledge it offers. Through the collective experiences of others, we gain insights, strategies, and resources that can enhance our healing journey. We learn from those who have walked the path before us, finding comfort in their guidance and knowing that we are not alone in our quest for liberation.

In community, we have the opportunity to lend our own support and encouragement to fellow warriors. By offering a listening ear, sharing our stories, and providing of wisdom, we become catalysts for transformation in the lives of others. In this act of giving, we discover the profound impact we can have on someone else's healing journey.

Community extends beyond the boundaries of physical proximity. It transcends geographical limitations and finds its home in the virtual realm. Online support groups, forums, and social media communities become platforms for connection and inspiration. Through these digital spaces, we can reach out to individuals from all walks of life, united by a common goal of healing and liberation.

The power of community lies not only in its ability to support individual healing but also in its potential to ignite collective change. As we come together, sharing our stories and raising awareness about Candida and sugar addiction, we create a ripple effectâ€"a wave of knowledge and empowerment that reaches far beyond our immediate circles. In this united effort, we become agents of change, challenging societal norms and advocating for greater understanding and support.

Embracing community also invites us to cultivate compassion for ourselves and others. It teaches us to celebrate the uniqueness of each individual's journey, recognizing that we are all at different stages and facing different challenges. Through compassion, we create an inclusive space that honors diversity and encourages growth and healing at our own pace.

Dear reader, as you embrace the power of community, remember that you are not alone on this journey. Reach out, connect, and allow yourself to be supported. In community, you will find strength, understanding, and the unwavering belief that healing is possible.

In the final chapters of our journey, we will explore the themes of resilience, transformation, and embracing a life of freedom beyond Candida and sugar addiction. Get ready to embark on the path of empowerment as we uncover the secrets to lasting change.

Chapter 11: Resilience: Rising from the Ashes of Adversity

: 1018

In the face of adversity and the grueling battle against Candida and sugar addiction, resilience emerges as a beacon of hope—a force that propels us forward and empowers us to rise from the ashes. Resilience is the ability to bounce back, to find strength amidst challenges, and to persevere in the face of setbacks.

Life's journey is often marked by unexpected twists and turns, and our healing journey is no exception. There may be times when we stumble, when the weight of the battle feels too heavy to bear. It is in these moments that resilience becomes our greatest ally—an unwavering companion that reminds us of our inner strength and fuels our determination to keep moving forward.

Resilience is not a trait that is solely bestowed upon a chosen few; it is a quality that can be cultivated and nurtured within each of us. It is a mindset—an unwavering belief that we have the capacity to overcome, to learn, and to grow from every experience. Resilience teaches us that setbacks are not the end, but an opportunity for growth and transformation.

In the face of Candida and sugar addiction, resilience asks us to shift our perspective and embrace the challenges as catalysts for change. It invites us to reframe our setbacks as stepping stones towards a healthier and more fulfilling life. With resilience as our guide, we navigate the intricate labyrinth of healing, knowing that each step forward, no matter how small, is a victory in itself.

Resilience is not about denying our pain or suppressing our emotions; it is about acknowledging them and allowing ourselves to feel. It is through the process of acceptance and self-compassion that we find the inner resilience to move forward. We honor our emotions, embracing them as messengers, and offering ourselves the love and support we need to heal.

One of the key elements of resilience is adaptabilityâ€"the ability to adjust and recalibrate our strategies in the face of new challenges. As we progress on our healing journey, we may encounter unexpected roadblocks or triggers that require us to adapt our approach. Resilience allows us to be flexible, to let go of rigidity, and to explore alternative paths towards our goals.

In the realm of self-care, resilience invites us to prioritize our well-being and set boundaries that protect our energy. It teaches us to listen to the whispers of our bodies, to honor our limitations, and to practice self-care as an act of resilience. We recognize that self-care is not selfish, but a vital component of our ability to show up fully and authentically in the world.

Resilience is not a solitary endeavor; it thrives in the embrace of community and support. The connections we forge with others on our healing journey become pillars of strength that bolster our resilience. Through sharing our stories, offering and receiving support, and celebrating our victories, we create a network of resilience that lifts us up during the most challenging times.

Dear reader, as you cultivate resilience on your healing journey, remember that you possess an inner strength that is unyielding. Trust in your ability to rise above the challenges, to learn from the setbacks, and to continue moving forward. Embrace the power of resilience and know that you are capable of creating a life of freedom and fulfillment beyond Candida and sugar addiction.

In the final chapters of our journey, we will explore the transformative power of embracing change and stepping into a life of liberation. Get ready to unleash your full potential as we unlock the secrets to lasting transformation.

Chapter 12: Embracing Change: Unlocking the Door to Freedom

: 1012

Change—a word that evokes a mix of anticipation, fear, and excitement. As we stand at the threshold of transformation in our battle against Candida and sugar addiction, embracing change becomes a gateway to freedom—a courageous step towards a life of liberation and renewed vitality.

Change is an inherent part of life's tapestryâ€"a constant rhythm that pulses through the very fabric of our existence. It is through change that growth and evolution become possible. In our healing journey, embracing change asks us to let go of old patterns, beliefs, and habits that no longer serve us. It invites us to open ourselves up to new possibilities and to embark on a path of self-discovery and transformation.

Embracing change requires courageâ€"the courage to step into the unknown, to confront our fears, and to challenge the familiar. It is in these moments of vulnerability and uncertainty that our true strength emerges. We find the resilience to face the discomfort and the determination to pursue a better and healthier life.

Change is not a linear process; it is a dance—a delicate interplay of surrender and action. It calls for patience and self-compassion as we navigate the ebb and flow of our healing journey. We allow ourselves to be guided by intuition, trusting that the path we are on is leading us towards our highest potential.

At times, change may feel like a storm—a whirlwind of emotions, doubts, and resistance. It is in these tempestuous moments that we lean into our inner strength and resilience. We remind ourselves of the vision we hold for our lives—a vision of vibrant health, inner peace, and a renewed sense of purpose. With each step forward, we reclaim our power and inch closer to the freedom we seek.

Embracing change also requires us to cultivate a mindset of curiosity and openness. We become explorers of our own inner landscape, unearthing hidden beliefs and patterns that have kept us trapped in the cycle of Candida and sugar addiction. Through self-reflection and self-awareness, we gain insights into the roots of our struggles and empower ourselves to create lasting change.

In the realm of our relationships, embracing change asks us to set boundaries and communicate our needs with clarity and compassion. We may encounter resistance from those who are accustomed to the old versions of ourselves. Yet, by staying true to our healing journey and honoring our growth, we inspire others to embark on their own paths of transformation.

Dear reader, as you embrace change, remember that you are not alone on this journey. Draw strength from the support of your community, from the wisdom of those who have walked this path before you, and from the unwavering belief in your own potential. Embrace change as an opportunity for growth, a catalyst for transformation, and a doorway to freedom.

In the final chapters of our journey, we will explore the culmination of our effortsâ€”the life of freedom and fulfillment that awaits us beyond Candida and sugar addiction. Get ready to step into the radiant light of liberation as we unlock the secrets to living a vibrant and empowered life.

Chapter 13: A Life Transformed: Radiating Freedom and Fulfillment

: 1005

As we near the culmination of our journey, we arrive at a pivotal momentâ€"a moment where the shackles of Candida and sugar addiction are shattered, and a life of freedom and fulfillment beckons us forward. It is a moment of profound transformationâ€"a rebirth of the spirit and a radiant awakening of the soul.

A life transformed is a life that knows no boundariesâ€"a life liberated from the chains of cravings, fatigue, and the limitations that once held us captive. It is a life where vibrant health, boundless energy, and inner peace converge in a symphony of joy and well-being. It is a life where we are the authors of our own destiny, reclaiming our power and embracing the limitless possibilities that lay before us.

In this new chapter of our lives, we rediscover the true essence of ourselvesâ€"the radiant beings that we were meant to be. We let go of the labels and judgments that have weighed us down, and we step into our authenticity with unwavering confidence. We embrace our uniqueness and celebrate the journey that has shaped us into the resilient warriors we have become.

A life transformed is not merely the absence of Candida and sugar addiction; it is the presence of a deep sense of purpose and fulfillment. We awaken to our passions, our gifts, and our innate talents, using them as beacons to guide us towards a life of meaning and contribution. We step into our power, knowing that our experiences have equipped us with wisdom and empathy to support others on their healing journeys.

In this transformed life, self-care becomes a sacred ritualâ€"a non-negotiable act of love and reverence for ourselves. We prioritize nourishing our bodies, minds, and spirits, recognizing that self-care is not a luxury but an essential foundation for our well-being. We listen to the whispers of our bodies, nurturing them with wholesome foods, movement, rest, and moments of quiet reflection.

Our relationships take on a new dimension in this transformed life. We surround ourselves with individuals who uplift and inspire us—those who see our potential and encourage us to soar. We cultivate deep connections built on trust, authenticity, and mutual support. We become pillars of strength for others, sharing our stories of triumph and offering a beacon of hope for those still on their journey towards liberation.

Gratitude infuses every fiber of our being in this transformed life. We appreciate the simple joys, the moments of connection, and the beauty that surrounds us. We recognize that each day is a precious gift, and we savor every breath, every smile, and every experience that comes our way. Gratitude becomes the fuel that ignites our passion and infuses our lives with a profound sense of fulfillment.

Dear reader, as we conclude our journey together, take a moment to reflect on how far you have come. Celebrate the resilience that has carried you through the challenges, and embrace the radiant light of transformation that now illuminates your path. Know that the life of freedom and fulfillment that awaits you is not a distant dream, but a tangible reality that you can create.

With your newfound wisdom, inner strength, and unwavering determination, step forward into this transformed life with open arms and a heart full of gratitude. Embrace the endless possibilities that await you, and know that you are destined to live a life of vibrant health, joy, and fulfillment beyond Candida and sugar addiction.

This is the beginning of a new chapterâ€"a chapter filled with limitless potential and infinite possibilities. Embrace it, dear reader, and let your transformed life unfold in all its brilliance.

Chapter 14: The Ripple Effect: Inspiring Change in Others

: 1012

As we bask in the radiance of our transformed lives, we come to realize that our journey extends far beyond our own personal liberation. We discover the profound power we hold to inspire change in othersâ€"to create a ripple effect that extends to every corner of the world.

Our transformation becomes a catalyst for transformation in those around us. Through our authenticity, resilience, and unwavering commitment to our well-being, we become beacons of hope, guiding others towards their own path of healing and liberation. We embody the living proof that change is possible, igniting a spark of possibility in the hearts of those who cross our path.

The ripple effect begins with the simple act of sharing our story—the story of our battle against Candida and sugar addiction, and the triumphs that have emerged from the depths of our struggle. Our vulnerability becomes a bridge of connection—a reminder to others that they are not alone in their own battles. We offer a compassionate ear, a safe space for them to share their fears, hopes, and dreams.

In sharing our story, we inspire others to embark on their own healing journeys. We plant seeds of curiosity and possibility, inviting them to question the status quo and to envision a life beyond the confines of their current struggles. We ignite the flame of hope, reminding them that they too possess the strength and resilience to overcome their challenges.

Our transformed lives serve as living testimonies to the power of self-care and self-love. As we prioritize our well-being and nourish our bodies, minds, and spirits, others witness the transformation that unfolds before their eyes. They see the radiance in our eyes, the vitality in our step, and the joy that emanates from our being. It is through this silent language of transformation that we inspire change in others.

By embracing our uniqueness and pursuing our passions, we give permission for others to do the same. We become catalysts for self-discovery and self-expression, encouraging others to explore their own interests, talents, and dreams. In doing so, we create a world where individuals are empowered to live authentically and to contribute their unique gifts to the collective tapestry of humanity.

The ripple effect of our transformed lives extends beyond our immediate circles. It permeates the larger community, the society we inhabit, and the world at large. Our actions inspire change on a systemic level, encouraging shifts in perceptions, policies, and practices related to health and well-being. We become advocates for change, raising awareness, and challenging the status quo, as we strive to create a world that nurtures and supports the holistic well-being of all.

Dear reader, as you embrace your role as an agent of change, remember that the ripple effect begins with you. Your transformed life has the power to ignite a spark of transformation in others, to inspire hope, and to create a wave of change that can reshape the world. Embrace this power with humility, compassion, and a deep sense of responsibility.

Celebrate the victories, both big and small, of those who are inspired by your journey. Be a source of encouragement and support, providing a guiding light for those who are navigating their own healing paths. Together, we can create a world where liberation and well-being are accessible to all, where the ripple effect of transformation knows no bounds.

In the final chapter of our journey, we will reflect on the lessons learned, the wisdom gained, and the infinite possibilities that lie ahead. Get ready to step into a future filled with purpose, impact, and the fulfillment of your deepest aspirations.

Chapter 15: Beyond Boundaries: A Future Filled with Possibility

: 1018

As we reach the conclusion of our transformative journey, we stand on the precipice of a future brimming with boundless potential and infinite possibilities. We have traversed the depths of struggle, embraced change with unwavering courage, and inspired transformation in ourselves and those around us. Now, it is time to envision the magnificent tapestry of our lives unfolding beyond the boundaries we once thought possible.

In this future, we transcend the limitations that once held us captive. We shed the remnants of doubt and fear, stepping into our power with a renewed sense of purpose and confidence. We understand that our journey towards vibrant health and freedom was never meant to be confined to a singular chapter in our lives. It is a lifelong commitmentâ€"an ever-unfolding adventure of self-discovery, growth, and evolution.

With each passing day, we continue to cultivate a deep love and reverence for ourselves. We recognize our inherent worthiness and embrace self-compassion as the guiding light that illuminates our path. We cherish the unique tapestry of strengths, talents, and passions that make us who we are, and we wholeheartedly embrace the journey of self-discovery that lies ahead.

In this future, our vibrant health becomes a pillar of strength that allows us to fully embrace life's wonders. We savor the simple joysâ€"a sunrise painting the sky with hues of gold, the laughter of loved ones, and the taste of nourishing foods that fuel our bodies and souls. We revel in the boundless energy that courses through our veins, empowering us to chase our dreams and make a positive impact in the world.

Our transformed lives become a source of inspiration for others, extending the ripple effect of change far and wide. We become catalysts for a collective awakeningâ€"an invitation for individuals from all walks of life to embark on their own journeys of healing, growth, and liberation. We create a world where the pursuit of vibrant health and holistic well-being is not a luxury but a fundamental human right.

In this future, we embrace the interconnectedness of all beings and the sacredness of our planet. We nurture a deep reverence for Mother Earth, recognizing that our well-being is intricately intertwined with the well-being of the natural world. We become stewards of the environment, tending to its beauty, protecting its resources, and working tirelessly to create a sustainable and harmonious future for generations to come.

As we gaze into the horizon of this future, we acknowledge that the path may not always be smooth. We may encounter obstacles and setbacks along the way. But armed with the resilience, wisdom, and unwavering determination we have cultivated throughout our journey, we face these challenges with grace and perseverance. We know that every stumbling block is an opportunity for growth, and every detour is a chance to recalibrate our course towards our highest potential.

Dear reader, as we bid farewell to this transformative journey, carry the lessons and experiences gained within your heart. Know that the possibilities that lie ahead are vast and wondrous. Trust in your innate wisdom, harness the power of your dreams, and walk forward with the unwavering belief that you have the capacity to create a future beyond your wildest imagination.

Embrace the beauty of the unknown, for it is within the uncharted territories that the most profound growth and transformation await. Embrace the truth that you are a beacon of light, a catalyst for change, and a living testament to the power of resilience, love, and self-belief.

As we close this chapter, remember that your journey towards vibrant health, freedom, and fulfillment is not the end but the beginningâ€"an eternal voyage of self-discovery, purpose, and the relentless pursuit of a life well-lived. Embrace the endless possibilities that await you, dear reader, and embark on this extraordinary adventure with open arms and a heart full of hope.

www.ingramcontent.com/pod-product-compliance
Lightning Source LLC
Chambersburg PA
CBHW050041260726
48658CB00005B/1713